# NATURAL FERTILITY HEALING BOOK

## Step By Step Guide On How To Cure Common Fertility Issues Naturally

Joyce Lifted

# COPYRIGHT

# Table of Contents

# WHO IS THIS BOOK FOR?

If you are not ready to get pregnant, please don't try to practices any of this remedy I shall mention in this book because is very active and you will actually get pregnant if not careful. So is strictly for couples who are struggling to conceive most especially women but they are unable due to few of the common reproductive issues or the other.

This natural fertility healing book is a comprehensive resource that provides guidance on how to optimize fertility naturally. These books typically cover a wide range of topics, including the role of nutrition in fertility, natural remedies for common reproductive issues, lifestyle changes that can enhance fertility, and strategies for managing stress and improving emotional well being.

# INTRODUCTION

Natural fertility healing is a topic of growing interest for couples who are struggling to conceive. For many people, the traditional medical approach to infertility may not be suitable, or they may simply prefer a more holistic approach to reproductive health. In recent years, there have been an increasing number of books and resources available that focus on natural fertility healing, providing guidance on diet, lifestyle, and natural remedies to enhance fertility. These books offer a wealth of knowledge and practical advice for those looking to improve their chances of conceiving naturally. In this introduction, we will explore the concept of natural fertility healing and discuss how a natural fertility healing book can be a valuable resource for anyone seeking to improve their reproductive health.

# CHAPTER 1

## CONCEPTS FOR NATURAL FERTILITY HEALING BOOK

Natural fertility healing is an approach to treating fertility issues that focuses on using natural methods to improve reproductive health and increase the chances of conception. This approach involves addressing underlying imbalances and deficiencies in the body that may be contributing to infertility, as well as supporting overall health and wellness.

There are several key concepts that underlie the natural fertility healing approach:

**Holistic approach**: Natural fertility healing takes a holistic approach to reproductive health, considering the body as a whole rather than focusing solely on the reproductive system. This approach recognizes that fertility is influenced by a range of factors, including diet, lifestyle, stress levels, and environmental exposures, and seeks to address imbalances in all of these areas.

**Individualized care:** Natural fertility healing recognizes that each person's body and fertility journey is unique. As such, treatment plans are tailored to each individual's specific needs and may involve a combination of dietary changes, lifestyle modifications, supplements, and other natural therapies.

**Addressing underlying imbalances**: Natural fertility healing focuses on identifying and addressing underlying imbalances in the body that may be contributing to fertility issues. This may include addressing hormonal imbalances, supporting proper thyroid function, improving gut health, and addressing inflammation.

## Here Are Some Common Fertility Issues That Affect Women

- Hormonal imbalances
- Ovulatory disorders
- Fallopian tube blockage

# CHAPTER 2

# THE ROLE OF NUTRITION IN FERTILITY

Some people neglect the role of nutrition in their well being and some are not even aware of what role its plays in fertility. Majority of the intake of nutrition in our body system is what causes most of the fertility issues we are suffering from especially in Africa. Nutrition plays an important role in fertility for both sex. A balanced and nutritious diet can positively impact reproductive health, hormone production, and overall fertility. Here are some key aspects of the role of nutrition in fertility:

1. **Healthy body weight:** Maintaining a healthy body weight is important for fertility. Both underweight and

overweight conditions can affect hormonal balance and disrupt the menstrual cycle in women. For men, obesity can lead to decreased sperm quality and quantity. A good balanced diet can help to achieve and maintain a healthy weight.

2. **Macronutrients:** Adequate intake of macronutrients, such as proteins, carbohydrates, and fats, is important for reproductive health. Proteins are essential for the production of reproductive hormones and egg/sperm development. Complex carbohydrates provide energy and fiber, while healthy fats (e.g., omega-3 fatty acids) support hormone production.

3. **Micronutrients:** Several micronutrients play critical roles in fertility. Some examples include:

**Folic acid**: Crucial for women planning to conceive, as it helps prevent neural tube defects in the fetus. Good sources include leafy green vegetables, beans, and fortified cereals.

**Iron:** Important for women to prevent anemia, which can affect fertility and pregnancy. Good sources include lean meats, poultry, fish, and legumes.

**Zinc:** Essential for both male and female fertility. It helps regulate hormone levels and supports healthy sperm production.

Good sources include oysters, lean meats, nuts, and seeds.

**Vitamin D:** Inadequate levels have been linked to infertility and hormonal imbalances. Natural sources include sunlight, fatty fish, and fortified dairy products.

4. **Antioxidants:** Antioxidants, such as vitamins C and E, selenium, and coenzyme Q10, help protect reproductive cells from oxidative stress and damage. They are found in fruits, vegetables, nuts, and seeds.

5. Omega-3 fatty acids: These healthy fats are known to improve fertility in both men and women. They can be

found in fatty fish (like salmon and sardines), flaxseeds, chia seeds, and walnuts.

6. **Hydration:** Staying hydrated is essential for maintaining healthy cervical mucus production in women and optimal sperm health in men.

7. **Avoiding harmful substances:** Limiting or avoiding alcohol, caffeine, smoking, and recreational drug use is important for fertility. These substances can negatively affect hormone levels, sperm quality, and reproductive health.

It's important to note that while nutrition plays a significant role in fertility, it's not the sole factor. Other factors like age, underlying medical conditions, genetics, and lifestyle choices also influence fertility. If you're facing challenges with fertility, it's advisable to consult a healthcare professional for personalized advice and guidance

# Chapter 3

## LIFESTYLE CHANGES THAT CAN ENHANCE FERTILITY

Making certain lifestyle changes can help enhance fertility. Here are some suggestions:

**Maintain a healthy weight**: Both being overweight and underweight can affect fertility. In other to have a healthy weight range, you must engage yourself in the following  balanced diet and also engage in regular physical activity.

**Eat a nutritious diet:** Consume a well-balanced diet rich in fruits, vegetables, whole grains, lean proteins, and healthy fats. Include foods that are high in antioxidants, such as berries, leafy greens, and nuts, as they may improve fertility.

**Avoid excessive alcohol and caffeine:** Limit your alcohol intake as it can decrease fertility. Additionally, high caffeine consumption has been associated with reduced fertility, so it's advisable to limit caffeine intake from sources like coffee, tea, and soda.

**Quit smoking:** Smoking has a detrimental impact on both male and female fertility. It can decrease sperm count, motility, and quality in males, while in females, it can affect egg quality and increase the risk of miscarriage. Quitting smoking is crucial for optimizing fertility.

**Exercise moderately**: Engage in regular physical activity, but avoid overexertion. Moderate exercise helps maintain a healthy weight, improves circulation, and reduces stress levels. However, excessive intense exercise may disrupt menstrual cycles and affect fertility.

Manage stress: High levels of stress can interfere with hormonal balance and affect fertility. Find stress-management techniques that work for you, such as exercise, yoga, meditation, or engaging in hobbies.

**Get enough sleep:** Prioritize quality sleep and aim for 7-9 hours of uninterrupted sleep each night. Proper rest is essential for hormonal regulation and overall well-being.

**Minimize exposure to toxins:** Reduce your exposure to environmental toxins, such as pesticides, chemicals, and pollutants. This includes avoiding certain household cleaning products, cosmetics with harmful ingredients, and exposure to secondhand smoke.

**Practice safe sex:** Protect yourself from sexually transmitted infections (STIs) by practicing safe sex. Certain STIs, if left untreated, can lead to infertility.

Seek regular medical check-ups:
Schedule routine check-ups with your healthcare provider to monitor your overall health and address any potential fertility concerns promptly.

Remember, while these lifestyle changes can enhance fertility for many individuals, infertility can be caused by various factors. If you're experiencing difficulties conceiving, it's recommended to consult with a healthcare professional or a fertility specialist for personalized advice and support.

# Chapter 3

## Hormonal Imbalance

**Introduction to hormonal imbalance and natural remedy to balance hormone**

Hormonal imbalance in females refers to an abnormality in the levels of hormones that regulate various bodily functions. Hormonal imbalances can affect fertility, increase the risk of certain cancers, and contribute to a range of health problems, including polycystic ovary syndrome (PCOS), endometriosis, thyroid disorders, and diabetes. Its occurs when there is much or little of one or more hormones in the bloodstream. A small hormonal imbalance can cause side effect in the body.

There are several possible causes of hormonal imbalance in females, which including the following below:

Age: Hormonal changes occur naturally during puberty, menopause, and per menopause.

Stress: Chronic stress can lead to imbalances in the stress hormone cortisol and other hormones.

Poor diet: Eating a diet high in processed foods, sugar, and unhealthy fats can contribute to hormonal imbalances.

Lack of exercise: A sedentary lifestyle can lead to imbalances in hormones that regulate metabolism and weight.

**Medications:** Certain medications such as birth control pills, hormone replacement therapy, and some psychiatric medications can affect hormone levels.

Underlying medical conditions: Conditions such as polycystic ovary syndrome (PCOS), thyroid disorders, and diabetes can lead to hormonal imbalances.

Environmental toxins: Exposure to toxins such as pesticides, plastics, and pollutants can disrupt the endocrine system and lead to hormonal imbalances.

## Symptoms of Hormonal Imbalance

**Irregular periods:** Changes in estrogen and progesterone levels can cause irregular menstrual cycles.

**Heavy or painful periods:** Imbalances in estrogen and progesterone can cause heavier and more painful periods.

**Hot flashes and night sweats:** A drop in estrogen levels during menopause can cause these symptoms.

**Mood swings:** Changes in hormone levels can affect mood and lead to irritability, anxiety, and depression.

**Weight gain:** Hormonal imbalances can cause changes in metabolism and lead to weight gain.

**Acne:** Fluctuations in hormones such as testosterone can cause acne. Hormonal imbalances can cause different types of acne, but the most common type is known as "hormonal acne". This type of acne typically appears along the jaw line, chin, and lower cheeks. Hormonal acne is usually caused by an increase in androgens (male hormones) such as testosterone, which stimulate the oil glands in the skin, leading to excess oil production and clogged pores.

Hormonal acne can appear as blackheads, whiteheads, papules, pustules, or cysts. It can be more severe than other types of acne and may be more resistant to treatment. Hormonal acne can also be triggered or exacerbated by certain factors such as stress, menstrual cycles, and certain medications.

**Hair loss**: Imbalances in thyroid hormones or androgens can cause hair loss.

**Fatigue:** Changes in hormone levels can cause fatigue and low energy levels.

**Reduced sex drive:** Changes in estrogen and testosterone levels can affect libido and lead to reduced sex drive.

# HOW TO CURE HORMONAL IMBALANCE THROUGH NATURAL USED OF HOME SUPPLEMENT

There are several natural ways and different ingredient used in balancing hormone. First let's get to lists out the ingredients used to balance your hormone naturally at home and their function in to human consumptions... And am going to list out other kinds of ingredient that you will be able to identify because I know is not all the ingredient you may know or identify depending on your locations.

**The ingredients and their functions are**:

- **Pineapple peel:** Pineapple peel can be useful in several ways like nutritional values, skin care, anti-inflammatory, digestive health etc.  Pineapple peel contains high amount fiber and enzymes that can help promote healthy digestion and prevent constipation.

- **Lemon orange**: Lemon is a versatile fruits that is rich with many useful properties such as vitamin c, digestion, hydration, and skin care and cleaning.
- **Cabbage:** cabbage is a versatile nutritious vegetable that has many useful properties which includes vital and useful properties, such as vitamin k, c and low calories.
- **Ginger:** Ginger has been used for centuries as a spice **and medicinal herb. It is well-known for its distinct** flavor and aroma, as well as its many health benefits. Here are some of the ways in which ginger can be useful:

**Reducing inflammation**: Ginger has compounds called gingerols and shogaols, which have anti-inflammatory properties.

These compounds help to reduce inflammation in the body and get rid of pain associated with conditions such as osteoarthritis and rheumatoid arthritis.

**Boosting immunity:** Ginger has antiviral, antibacterial, and antioxidant properties, which can help boost the immune system and prevent illness.

**Improving digestion:** Ginger can stimulate digestion and help relieve digestive problems such as bloating, gas, and constipation.

**Lowering cholesterol:** Some studies have shown that ginger can help lower cholesterol levels and reduce the risk of heart disease.

**Fighting infections:** Ginger has natural antibiotic properties, which can help fight off infections and promote overall health.

- **Cloves:** cloves have many potential health benefits that are useful to the body.

**Relieving pain:** Cloves contain a compound called eugenol, which has analgesic properties. This means that cloves can help alleviate pain, particularly toothaches and headaches.

**Improving digestion:** Cloves can stimulate digestion and help relieve digestive problems such as bloating, gas, and constipation. They also have antispasmodic properties, which can help soothe the muscles of the digestive tract and alleviate cramping.

**Boosting the immune system:** Cloves have antiviral, antibacterial, and anti-inflammatory properties, which can help boost the immune system and prevent illness.

Controlling blood sugar: Some studies have shown that cloves can help regulate blood sugar levels, which is beneficial for people with diabetes.

Supporting oral health: The eugenol in cloves also has antiseptic properties, which can help kill bacteria in the mouth and prevent gum disease and bad breath.

Improving respiratory health: Cloves contain compounds that can help alleviate respiratory problems such as coughs, colds, and asthma...

- Cinnamon: Cinnamon is a popular spice that is used in cooking and baking, and it also has several potential health benefits. Here are some ways in which cinnamon sticks or powder can be useful:

**Controlling blood sugar:** Cinnamon contains compounds that can help regulate blood sugar levels, making it a useful spice for people with diabetes or those at risk of developing diabetes.

**Lowering cholesterol**: Some studies have shown that cinnamon can help lower LDL (bad) cholesterol and triglycerides, which can help reduce the risk of heart disease.

**Anti-inflammatory properties**: Cinnamon contains compounds with anti-inflammatory properties, which can help reduce inflammation in the body and alleviate pain associated with conditions such as arthritis.

**Boosting the immune system:** Cinnamon has antimicrobial, antiviral, and antibacterial properties, which can help boost the immune system and prevent illness.

**Improving cognitive function**: Some studies have suggested that cinnamon may have cognitive benefits, such as improving memory and attention span.

**Reducing the risk of cancer:** Cinnamon contains compounds that have shown to inhibit the growth of cancer cells in some studies.

So you can see that all this ingredients listed above are rich in fiber, they all have low calories, they are immune booster, rich in vitamin c, and K. And secondly these ingredients have been used by several people and it works for them. So don't be afraid about it.

## Procedure

STEP 1: wash the pineapple peel and dice them to smaller portion into a clean pot

STEP 2: wash the cabbage and dice them too into small portion then pour it into the same pot you put the pineapple peels.

STEP 3: peel out the bark of the ginger and wash it in clean water, thereafter you slice the ginger and still pour it into the same pot.

STEP 3: wash the remaining ingredients and cut them to smaller portions then pour all of them into the same pot

STEP 4: pours in 2liters of water into the pot, note and remember that the quantity of water you pour into the pot determined the quantity of the substance in the pot.

STEP 5: boil it for 15mins and take it down, then filter it to another container and make it cold for drinking. Drink one glass cup of it morning with an empty stomach and one glass cup of it at night before you sleep.

Drink this for two weeks and the hormonal imbalance will be cure.

# CHAPTER 4

## OVULATORY DISORDER

An ovulatory disorder refers to a condition in which a woman experiences irregular or absent ovulation, which can affect her ability to conceive or maintain a pregnancy. Ovulation is the process in which the ovaries release a mature egg that can be fertilized by sperm. When ovulation is disrupted or does not occur regularly, it can lead to difficulties in achieving pregnancy.

There are several types of ovulatory disorders, including:

Anovulation: This occurs when the ovaries do not release an egg during the menstrual cycle. Anovulation can be caused by hormonal imbalances, such as high levels of androgens (male hormones) or low levels of certain hormones like luteinizing hormone (LH) or follicle-stimulating hormone (FSH).

Polycystic ovary syndrome (PCOS): PCOS is a common hormonal disorder in women of reproductive age. It is characterized by the formation of small cysts on the ovaries, hormonal imbalances, and irregular ovulation or Anovulation. Women with PCOS may experience symptoms such as irregular periods, excessive hair growth, acne, and weight gain.

Hypothalamic dysfunction: The hypothalamus is a part of the brain that regulates the production of hormones involved in ovulation. Disruptions or abnormalities in the hypothalamus can lead to ovulatory disorders. Factors such as excessive exercise, extreme weight loss or gain, stress, or certain medical conditions can affect hypothalamic function.

Premature ovarian insufficiency (POI): Also known as premature ovarian failure, POI refers to the loss of normal ovarian function before the age of 40. Women with POI may have irregular or absent periods, decreased ovarian hormone production, and reduced fertility.

## Symptoms of ovulatory disorder

The symptom of ovulatory disorder depends on the causes and the symptoms includes;

Irregular menstrual cycles: Women with ovulatory disorders may experience irregular periods, meaning their menstrual cycles are unpredictable in terms of timing, duration, or flow.

Absent or infrequent periods: Some women may have very long gaps between their periods or even skip periods altogether due to lack of ovulation.

Abnormal bleeding: Ovulatory disorders can cause abnormal bleeding patterns, such as heavy or prolonged menstrual bleeding or spotting between periods.

Hormonal imbalances: Hormonal fluctuations associated with ovulatory disorders can lead to symptoms like acne, oily skin, changes in libido (sex drive), breast tenderness, or mood swings.

Changes in cervical mucus: Ovulation is often accompanied by changes in the consistency and appearance of cervical mucus. Women with ovulatory disorders may notice a lack of fertile cervical mucus or changes that deviate from the typical ovulatory pattern.

Pelvic pain: Some women with ovulatory disorders may experience pelvic pain or discomfort during or around the time of ovulation. This is known as mittelschmerz. The word Mittelschmerz is a German word that translates to "middle pain" or "pain in the middle." It refers to the abdominal or pelvic pain that some women experience during ovulation. Mittelschmerz typically occurs midway through the menstrual cycle, around the time when the ovary releases an egg.

The exact cause of mittelschmerz is not fully understood, but it is believed to be related to the stretching or irritation of the ovarian surface at the time of ovulation. As the egg is released from the ovary, a small amount of fluid or blood may be released as well, which can cause mild discomfort or pain in the lower abdomen on the side of the ovulating ovary.

The pain associated with mittelschmerz is typically described as sharp, cramp-like, or twinge-like. It may last anywhere from a few minutes to a few hours, but in some cases, it can persist for a day or two. The intensity of the pain can vary from mild to severe, and it may occur on one side of the lower abdomen or alternate sides from cycle to cycle.

Difficulty conceiving: Ovulatory disorders can significantly impact fertility and make it challenging for women to conceive. If a woman is actively trying to get pregnant and experiencing difficulty, it may be a sign of an ovulatory disorder.

# CAUSES OF OVULATORY DISORDER

There are various causes of ovulatory disorders, which can disrupt or prevent the regular release of eggs from the ovaries. Some common causes include:

**Hormonal Imbalances:** Hormonal imbalances are a significant factor in ovulatory disorders. Disruptions in the normal levels of hormones involved in the menstrual cycle, such as follicle-stimulating hormone (FSH), luteinizing hormone (LH), estrogen, and progesterone, can interfere with the maturation and release of eggs.

**Polycystic Ovary Syndrome (PCOS):** PCOS is a hormonal disorder that affects the ovaries and is one of the leading causes of ovulatory disorders. In PCOS, the ovaries may develop multiple small cysts and produce higher levels of androgens (male hormones) than normal. These hormonal imbalances can disrupt ovulation.

**Thyroid Disorders:** Thyroid dysfunction, such as hypothyroidism (underactive thyroid) or hyperthyroidism (overactive thyroid), can disrupt the normal hormonal balance in the body, leading to ovulatory disorders.

**Hypothalamic Dysfunction**: The hypothalamus is an area of the brain that plays a crucial role in regulating the menstrual cycle and ovulation. Conditions that affect the hypothalamus, such as excessive exercise, extreme weight loss or gain, chronic stress, or disorders like hypothalamic amenorrhea, can disrupt the hormonal signals necessary for ovulation.

**Premature Ovarian Insufficiency (POI):** Also known as premature ovarian failure, POI refers to the loss of normal ovarian function before the age of 40. This condition can be caused by genetic factors, autoimmune disorders, chemotherapy or radiation therapy, or certain infections. POI can result in irregular or absent ovulation.

**Other Medical Conditions**: Certain medical conditions, such as polyps or fibroids in the uterus, endometriosis, ovarian cysts, or structural abnormalities of the reproductive organs, can interfere with ovulation.

**Medications and Hormonal Birth Control**: Some medications, including certain antidepressants and antipsychotics, can affect hormonal balance and disrupt ovulation. Similarly, certain hormonal contraceptives, such as some types of birth control pills or long-acting reversible contraceptives (IUDs), can temporarily suppress ovulation.

# HOME INGREDIENTS REMEDY FOR PCOS

1. Groundnut(fresh groundnut with the chaff)
2. Cinnamon
3. Water

# Procedure on how to use the ingredients

Pound or blend a cup of groundnut daily, boil it with one and half cup of water for 8mins, after boiling it, add one table spoon of cinnamon powder, keep it to cool before you drink it. Drink it with the chaff once daily starting from the day you are suppose to see your ovulation for 14days and you will be surprise to see the result. Another simple home remedy for ovulation disorders are as follows;

1. Five finger of fresh okra
2. Cloves
3. Cinnamon stick or powder
4. Fresh groundnut with the chaff.

## Procedure

Slice the okra into a container and mix it with water, then cover it and keep for the next 24hrs.

Wash the cinnamon stick and put it in a plastic bottle, pour in the cloves together in the plastic bottle and add water to it, then cover it and keep it for 24hrs. When is 24hrs, you will filter the water okra into a glass cup, pour in your cinnamon water a little into the okra water and drink it. Then get ready to see the result. Note; you are to drink it in the morning in an empty stomach and also at night.

**How long should I drink this?**
Drink it for 5 days
**When should I drink it?**
Drink it immediately after your menstruation.

Or if you can't find some of this ingredients, you can used only the okra water, but you must soak the okra in the water for 24 hrs, and make sure you drink it immediately after your menstruation, that is, if your menstruation is finishing today, you must prepare the recipes the day before your last flow and start drinking it the day after your last flow. Please take it in the morning and at night. This remedy can give you twins because is going to make you to hyper ovulate.

# Chapter 5
## Fallopian Tube Blockage
A Brief Introduction and Definition of Fallopian Tube Blockage

Fallopian tube blockage refers to the condition where one or both of the fallopian tubes, also known as uterine tubes or oviducts, are partially or completely obstructed. The fallopian tubes are a pair of narrow, muscular tubes that connect the ovaries to the uterus in the female reproductive system. They play a crucial role in facilitating the transport of eggs from the ovaries to the uterus and providing a site for fertilization to occur.

When the fallopian tubes become blocked, it can disrupt the normal movement of eggs, sperm, and fertilized embryos, leading to fertility problems. The blockage can occur at different points along the fallopian tubes, such as the proximal end near the uterus or the distal end close to the ovaries. The blockage can be caused by various factors, including infections, inflammatory conditions, endometriosis, previous surgeries, or congenital abnormalities. Identifying and addressing the underlying cause of the blockage is essential for effective management and potential restoration of fertility.

# Importance of Fallopian Tubes in Female Reproductive System

The fallopian tubes play an important role in the female reproductive system.  And the important are:

Egg Transport: The primary function of the fallopian tubes is to transport eggs (ova) from the ovaries to the uterus. After ovulation, when an egg is released from the ovary, it is captured by the fimbriae (finger-like projections at the end of the fallopian tubes) and guided into the fallopian tube. The tubes provide a pathway for the egg to travel towards the uterus.

Site of Fertilization: Fertilization is the union of sperm and egg typically occurs within the fallopian tubes. Sperm cells introduced through intercourse or assisted reproductive techniques, travel through the cervix, uterus, and into the fallopian tubes, where they can encounter and fertilize the egg. The fallopian tubes create a conducive environment for fertilization to take place.

Embryo Transport: Once fertilization occurs, the resulting embryo starts dividing and forms into a ball of cells called a blastocyst. The fallopian tubes help facilitate the movement of the developing embryo from the site of fertilization in the tube's ampulla (widest portion) toward the uterus. The tube's muscular contractions and the cilia lining its walls assist in this transportation process.

Nourishment and Development: As the embryo travels through the fallopian tubes, it receives nourishment from the surrounding fluids and gains the necessary conditions for early development. The tubes provide an optimal environment for the embryo's initial stages, including cell division and early differentiation.

Protection against Infection: The fallopian tubes act as a barrier, preventing harmful bacteria and other pathogens from entering the uterus and potentially causing infections. The tubes produce secretions that help maintain a healthy environment and prevent microbial colonization.

Overall, the fallopian tubes are essential for successful reproduction.

# Causes of Fallopian Tube Blockage

Pelvic Inflammatory Disease (PID): Pelvic Inflammatory Disease is the most common causes of fallopian tube blockage in women. It is an infection of that take place in the reproductive organs, usually caused by sexually transmitted infections (STIs) like Chlamydia or gonorrhea. The infection can lead to inflammation and scarring of the fallopian tubes, resulting in blockages.

Endometriosis: Endometriosis is a condition in which the tissue lining the uterus (endometrium) grows outside the uterus, commonly on the fallopian tubes, ovaries, or pelvic organs. The abnormal tissue growth can cause adhesions and blockages in the fallopian tubes.

Previous Surgeries or Ectopic Pregnancies: Surgeries involving the reproductive organs, such as surgeries to remove ovarian cysts or to treat ectopic pregnancies (implantation of a fertilized egg outside the uterus), can cause scarring or damage to the fallopian tubes, leading to blockages.

Uterine Fibroids or Polyps: Uterine fibroids are non-cancerous growths that can develop in or around the uterus. Depending on their location, fibroids can distort or block the fallopian tubes. Similarly, uterine polyps (small, benign growths on the uterine lining) can obstruct the fallopian tubes.

Congenital Abnormalities: Some individuals may be born with structural abnormalities in their fallopian tubes that can result in blockages. These abnormalities can include a complete absence of the tubes (congenital absence of the fallopian tubes) or abnormal shapes that hinder the passage of eggs or sperm.

Other Factors: Other potential causes of fallopian tube blockage include adhesions or scar tissue formation due to previous surgeries, pelvic infections unrelated to PID or certain conditions like tubal ligation (surgical sterilization) where the tubes are intentionally blocked.

# Symptoms of fallopian tube blockage

Infertility: The most significant symptom of fallopian tube blockage is difficulty conceiving or infertility. If the fallopian tubes are partially or completely blocked, it can hinder the movement of sperm towards the egg and prevent the fertilized egg from reaching the uterus for implantation.

Pelvic Pain: Some individuals with fallopian tube blockage may experience intermittent or chronic pelvic pain. The pain can range from mild discomfort to severe cramping and may be felt on one or both sides of the lower abdomen.

Abnormal Menstrual Bleeding: Blockages in the fallopian tubes can disrupt the normal menstrual cycle and cause changes in menstrual bleeding patterns. This can manifest as heavier or lighter periods, irregular periods, or spotting between periods.

Painful Intercourse: Sexual intercourse can be painful for individuals with fallopian tube blockage, especially if the pain is related to the inflammation or adhesions associated with the blockage.

Symptoms of Underlying Conditions: In some cases, the underlying conditions that contribute to fallopian tube blockage, such as pelvic during urination, or pain during bowel movements. Inflammatory disease (PID) or endometriosis, may present with additional symptoms like abnormal vaginal discharge, fever, pain.

## Treatments

Here is the natural treatment to unblock fallopian tube yourself by using this natural ingredients. The ingredients are;

1. Kola nut root
2. Quaver leaves
3. Water

## Procedure

1. Wash the quaver leaves and kola nut root thoroughly in a clean water,
2. Put the two ingredients in the pot and add water inside
3. Boil it for one hour

4. Drink the water as tea twice daily for two weeks and the fallopian tube blockage will melt away.

# CONCLUSION

This book serves as a comprehensive resource that empowers readers to make positive changes and embark on a path towards natural fertility healing. With the knowledge gained from this book, readers can better understand their bodies, nurture their overall well-being, and increase their chances of achieving the dream of parenthood.